THE PHILOSOPHY OF HAIDONG GUMDO

A Journey Towards Mastery: From Basic Principles to Advanced Techniques

KAMERON JALEN

Table of Contents

Introduction

Haidong Gumdo is a traditional Korean martial art that focuses on sword techniques and the philosophy of the warrior spirit. Haidong Gumdo was developed in the late 20th century, with its roots tracing back to ancient Korean swordsmanship practices. It was officially established in 1990. "Haidong" refers to the eastern sea, reflecting Korea's geographical location, while "Gumdo" means "the way of the sword."

Philosophy and Principles:

• **Martial Spirit**: Haidong Gumdo emphasizes not just physical skills but also the mental and spiritual aspects of martial arts. Practitioners are encouraged to cultivate discipline, respect, and humility.

• **Connection to Nature**: The practice often involves meditation and a deep appreciation for nature, aligning the practitioner's spirit with the environment.

Techniques and Training:

• **Sword Techniques**: The art includes a variety of sword techniques, such as cuts, thrusts, and parries. Practitioners learn through forms (hyung) and sparring (daeryun).

• **Training Methods**: Training involves not only practicing techniques but also strength and flexibility exercises, meditation, and breath control to enhance focus and precision.

Competitions and Demonstrations:

• **Tournaments**: Haidong Gumdo features competitive events where practitioners demonstrate their skills in forms and sparring.

• **Demonstrations**: High-level practitioners often showcase their abilities in public demonstrations, which may include breaking boards or performing choreographed routines.

Global Presence:

• **International Reach**: Since its inception, Haidong Gumdo has spread internationally, with schools and practitioners around the world. Organizations exist to promote its practice and philosophy globally.

Haidong Gumdo is more than just a martial art; it's a way of life that fosters physical fitness, mental discipline, and a connection to one's cultural heritage. Through the practice of sword techniques, practitioners strive to develop their skills while embodying the values of respect, humility, and perseverance.

Philosophy And Principles Of Haidong Gumdo

The philosophy and principles of Haidong Gumdo are integral to its practice, shaping not only the technical aspects but also the mindset and character of its practitioners. Here are the key elements of its philosophy and principles:

1. Warrior Spirit (Gumdo Shin):

• **Mindset**: Practitioners are encouraged to develop a warrior spirit, which encompasses qualities such as courage, honor, and resilience. This mindset helps practitioners face challenges both on and off the mat.

• **Discipline**: Training in Haidong Gumdo requires dedication and perseverance, fostering a sense of self-discipline that extends into everyday life.

2. Respect and Etiquette:

• **Hierarchical Structure**: Respect for instructors, seniors, and fellow practitioners is paramount. This is reflected in the formal etiquette observed during training, such as bowing and addressing others appropriately.

• **Cultural Heritage**: Practitioners learn to respect the traditions and history of Korean martial arts, ensuring that they honor the cultural significance of their training.

3. Harmony with Nature:

• **Connection to Nature**: The philosophy emphasizes a deep respect for nature and the environment. Practitioners are encouraged to find balance and harmony with the natural world, reflecting this in their movements and mindset.

• **Meditation and Awareness**: Mindfulness practices, including meditation and breath control, are used to cultivate awareness and foster a peaceful state of mind.

4. Holistic Development:

• **Physical and Mental Growth**: Haidong Gumdo promotes the development of both the body and mind. While mastering sword techniques is essential, practitioners also work on mental clarity, emotional stability, and spiritual growth.

• **Lifelong Learning**: The journey in Haidong Gumdo is seen as a continuous process of self-improvement and learning, encouraging practitioners to embrace challenges as opportunities for growth.

5. Integrity and Honor:

• **Moral Conduct**: Practitioners are expected to uphold high ethical standards and act with integrity. This includes using their skills responsibly and only in appropriate situations, promoting peace rather than conflict.

• **Community Engagement**: Haidong Gumdo encourages practitioners to contribute positively to their communities and to embody the values of compassion and support for others.

6. Mind-Body Connection:

• **Focus and Concentration**: Emphasis is placed on developing focus and concentration, allowing practitioners to perform techniques with precision and intention. This connection is cultivated through rigorous training and mindfulness practices.

• **Balance and Control**: Practitioners learn to achieve physical balance and control over their movements, reflecting a deeper understanding of their bodies and capabilities.

The philosophy and principles of Haidong Gumdo extend beyond physical techniques, encompassing a holistic approach to martial arts that nurtures the mind, body, and spirit. Practitioners strive to embody these values in their training and daily lives, fostering a sense of community and respect while pursuing personal growth and development.

The Role Of Meditation And Mindfulness

Meditation and mindfulness play a vital role in Haidong Gumdo, enhancing both the physical and mental aspects of the practice. Here's a closer look at how these elements are integrated into the martial art:

1. Mental Clarity and Focus:

• **Enhancing Concentration**: Regular meditation helps practitioners develop better focus and concentration, essential for executing precise techniques and forms. By quieting the mind, practitioners can direct their attention to their movements and the present moment.

• **Reducing Distractions**: Mindfulness practice encourages individuals to become aware of their thoughts and feelings without judgment, reducing mental clutter and allowing for a more centered training experience.

2. Stress Relief and Emotional Balance:

- **Managing Stress**: The practice of mindfulness can help alleviate stress and anxiety, making it easier for practitioners to remain calm and composed during training and competitions. This emotional stability contributes to better performance.

- **Cultivating Resilience**: Meditation fosters emotional awareness, enabling practitioners to navigate challenges and setbacks with a balanced mindset, promoting resilience in both martial arts and daily life.

3. Connection to the Present Moment:

- **Living in the Now**: Mindfulness encourages practitioners to engage fully in their training and experiences, helping them appreciate the process of learning and self-improvement. This connection to the present moment enhances the overall quality of practice.

- **Awareness of Movement**: Practicing mindfulness during training helps individuals become more attuned to their movements, improving their technique and efficiency in executing sword forms and techniques.

4. Spiritual Development:

- **Inner Peace**: Meditation practices often focus on cultivating inner peace and a sense of tranquility. This spiritual aspect aligns with the overall philosophy of Haidong Gumdo, which emphasizes harmony and balance.

- **Reflection and Growth**: Regular meditation provides time for self-reflection, allowing practitioners to assess their progress, set goals, and connect with their personal values and motivations in martial arts.

5. Enhancing Physical Performance:

• **Breath Control**: Mindful breathing techniques are crucial in both meditation and martial arts practice. Proper breath control enhances stamina, helps regulate energy levels, and improves overall performance during training.

• **Mind-Body Connection**: Meditation fosters a stronger mind-body connection, allowing practitioners to move more fluidly and intuitively, enhancing their overall martial arts skills.

6. Community and Connection:

• **Group Meditation**: Many Haidong Gumdo schools incorporate group meditation sessions, fostering a sense of community and shared purpose among practitioners. This collective experience enhances camaraderie and support within the martial arts community.

• **Shared Values**: The principles of mindfulness and meditation align with the core values of respect, integrity, and honor in Haidong Gumdo, strengthening the bonds among practitioners.

Meditation and mindfulness are essential components of Haidong Gumdo, contributing to the holistic development of practitioners. By fostering mental clarity, emotional balance, and a deep connection to the present moment, these practices enhance both the martial and personal aspects of training. As practitioners embrace meditation and mindfulness, they cultivate a more profound understanding of themselves and their journey in martial arts.

CHAPTER 1: FUNDAMENTAL CONCEPTS

Basic Terminology

Understanding the basic terminology of Haidong Gumdo is essential for practitioners and newcomers alike. Here are some key terms commonly used in the practice:

1. Gumdo (검도):

• **Translation**: "The Way of the Sword." This term refers to the martial art itself and encompasses its techniques, philosophy, and practices.

2. Hyung (형):

• **Translation**: "Form." These are predefined sequences of movements that practitioners learn and practice to develop their techniques, timing, and precision.

3. Daeryun (대련):

• **Translation**: "Sparring." This is the practice of engaging in controlled combat with a partner, allowing practitioners to apply their techniques in a dynamic environment.

4. Gum (검):

• **Translation**: "Sword." This term refers to the primary weapon used in Haidong Gumdo training. Practitioners learn various techniques involving the sword.

5. Chamber (참고):

• **Translation**: "To chamber." This refers to the position of the sword before executing a technique. Proper chambering is crucial for effective movement.

6. Kihap (기합):

• **Translation**: "Spirit shout." This is a loud shout made during training or competitions to focus energy, intimidate opponents, and enhance the practitioner's mental state.

7. Bodo (보도):

• **Translation**: "Sword techniques." This term encompasses the various cutting, thrusting, and defensive techniques taught in Haidong Gumdo.

8. Joonbi (준비);

• **Translation**: "Ready position." This is the stance practitioners take at the beginning of a form or sparring match, signaling readiness to engage.

9. Chireugi (치르기):

• **Translation**: "Cutting." This refers to the action of executing a cut with the sword, a fundamental aspect of Haidong Gumdo training.

10. Bong (봉):

• **Translation**: "Staff." In some schools, practitioners also train with a staff as an additional weapon, teaching skills that can complement sword techniques.

11. Seon (선):

• **Translation**: "Meditation." This term emphasizes the mental aspect of practice, where practitioners focus on mindfulness and awareness.

12. Dojang (도장):

• **Translation**: "Training hall." This is the place where practitioners train and practice Haidong Gumdo.

13. Saabum (사범):

• **Translation**: "Instructor." This term is used to refer to a qualified teacher or master in Haidong Gumdo.

14. Dan (단):

• **Translation**: "Degree." This refers to the ranking system in Haidong Gumdo, with various levels (typically colored belts) indicating a practitioner's proficiency.

These terms form the foundation of the vocabulary used in Haidong Gumdo. Familiarity with this terminology will enhance your understanding of the practice, making it easier to learn techniques, engage with instructors, and participate in training sessions.

Stances And Postures

In Haidong Gumdo, stances and postures are fundamental to effective sword techniques and overall martial arts practice. Each stance serves a specific purpose, aiding in balance, power generation, and readiness for action. Here are some of the key stances and postures used in Haidong Gumdo:

1. Joonbi Sogi (준비 자세) - Ready Stance:

• **Description**: This is the starting position for many forms and techniques. The feet are shoulder-width apart, and the sword is held with both hands, typically positioned at the waist or in front of the body.

• **Purpose**: It signals readiness to begin and allows for quick transitions into other movements.

2. Gum Sogi (검 자세) - Sword Stance:

• **Description**: In this stance, the sword is held in a high position, either over the shoulder or extended in front of the body.

• **Purpose**: It prepares the practitioner for both offensive and defensive actions, providing a strong and balanced posture for strikes.

3. Bandae Sogi (반대 자세) - Reverse Stance:

• **Description**: This stance involves turning the body to one side, with one foot positioned forward and the opposite foot back. The sword is often held in front for defense or ready to strike.

• **Purpose**: It enables quick movement and counterattacks, allowing the practitioner to pivot and change direction effectively.

4. Seong Sogi (성 자세) - Forward Stance:

• **Description**: The feet are positioned wide apart, with one foot forward and the other back. The front knee is bent, and the back leg is straight, providing stability and power.

• **Purpose**: This stance is used for powerful forward strikes and maintaining balance while delivering attacks.

5. Ninja Sogi (닌자 자세) - Low Stance:

• **Description**: This stance involves crouching low to the ground, with one knee bent and the other leg extended. The sword may be held low or ready for a quick thrust.

• **Purpose**: It allows for stealthy movement and quick transitions to attacks or evasive actions.

6. Charyot Sogi (차렷 자세) - Attention Stance:

• **Description**: In this stance, practitioners stand with feet together, hands at their sides or in front of the body. It is a formal posture used during ceremonies and respect.

• **Purpose**: This position signifies respect, focus, and discipline, often observed when entering or exiting the training hall.

7. Dwi Sogi (뒤 자세) - Back Stance:

• **Description**: This stance has the body turned slightly to the side, with the back leg bearing most of the weight. The sword is typically held at the hip or positioned for defense.

• **Purpose**: It prepares the practitioner for defensive maneuvers and allows for swift movement in any direction.

8. Dae Sogi (대 자세) - Wide Stance:

• **Description**: The feet are placed wider than shoulder-width, with the knees slightly bent. The body remains low and stable, with the sword positioned for defense or attack.

• **Purpose**: This stance provides a strong base for powerful cuts and defensive techniques, making it difficult for opponents to unbalance the practitioner.

9. Hui Sogi (희 자세) - Relaxed Stance:

• **Description**: This is a relaxed stance with feet shoulder-width apart, allowing for natural movement and breathing. The sword may be held loosely at the side or in front.

• **Purpose**: It promotes relaxation and awareness, serving as a transitional position between movements.

The various stances and postures in Haidong Gumdo are essential for executing techniques effectively and maintaining balance and control. Practicing these stances helps practitioners develop a strong foundation for their martial arts journey, enhancing their overall skill and adaptability in both training and sparring.

The Importance Of Breathing

Breathing is a fundamental aspect of Haidong Gumdo, playing a crucial role in enhancing performance, mental focus, and overall well-being. Here are the key reasons why proper breathing is important in this martial art:

1. Energy Management:

- **Breath Control**: Practitioners learn to control their breath to manage energy levels during training and sparring. Proper breathing techniques help conserve stamina, allowing for sustained performance over longer periods.

- **Qi (Chi) Flow**: In traditional martial arts, breath is often associated with the flow of vital energy (Qi). Practitioners aim to align their breathing with their movements to cultivate and direct this energy effectively.

2. Focus and Concentration:

• **Mental Clarity**: Controlled breathing enhances mental clarity and focus, allowing practitioners to concentrate on their movements and techniques without distractions. This heightened awareness is essential for effective execution during forms and sparring.

• **Mindfulness Practice**: Breathing techniques are integral to mindfulness practices in Haidong Gumdo, promoting a state of present-moment awareness that enhances overall training effectiveness.

3. Stress Reduction:

• **Relaxation Response**: Deep, controlled breathing activates the body's relaxation response, reducing stress and anxiety. This is particularly beneficial before competitions or intense training sessions, helping practitioners remain calm and centered.

• **Emotional Regulation**: Proper breathing can help practitioners manage their emotions, enabling them to stay composed during challenging situations and respond effectively rather than react impulsively.

4. Power Generation:

• **Kihap (Spirit Shout)**: In Haidong Gumdo, practitioners often incorporate a kihap, or spirit shout, with their breath during strikes. This explosive exhalation helps to generate power, creating a stronger impact during cuts and thrusts.

• **Breath Coordination**: Coordinating breath with movement enhances the force and precision of techniques. Inhalation and exhalation should be timed with specific movements to maximize effectiveness.

5. Physical Conditioning:

• **Endurance Training**: Practicing breath control during physical conditioning helps improve cardiovascular fitness and overall endurance. This is especially important for maintaining performance levels during long training sessions or competitions.

• **Recovery**: Proper breathing techniques aid in recovery by promoting relaxation and oxygenating the body after intense physical exertion. This facilitates quicker recovery and reduces fatigue.

6. Posture and Alignment:

• **Core Engagement**: Proper breathing encourages engagement of the core muscles, which helps maintain stability and proper alignment during techniques. This is vital for both balance and the execution of powerful movements.

- **Alignment Awareness**: Focusing on breath during training helps practitioners become more aware of their posture and alignment, leading to improved technique and reduced risk of injury.

7. Meditative Aspects;

- **Meditation Integration**: Breathing is central to meditation practices in Haidong Gumdo, helping practitioners cultivate a sense of inner peace and mindfulness. This meditative aspect enhances the overall training experience and personal growth.

The importance of breathing in Haidong Gumdo cannot be overstated. It is a key element that influences energy management, mental focus, emotional balance, power generation, and overall performance. By mastering breath control, practitioners can enhance their martial arts skills while promoting physical and mental well-being.

Principles Of Movement

The principles of movement in Haidong Gumdo are fundamental to executing techniques effectively and efficiently. These principles emphasize balance, coordination, and fluidity, enabling practitioners to perform sword techniques with power and precision. Here are some key principles of movement in Haidong Gumdo:

1. Balance:

• **Stability**: Maintaining a stable center of gravity is essential for effective movement. Practitioners learn to position their feet properly to ensure balance during both offensive and defensive maneuvers.

• **Weight Distribution**: Proper weight distribution between the feet allows for quick transitions between stances and movements, enabling practitioners to respond effectively to changing situations.

2. Flow and Fluidity:

• **Seamless Transitions**: Movement should be fluid and continuous, allowing practitioners to transition smoothly between techniques and stances. This flow enhances the overall effectiveness of techniques and helps maintain momentum.

• **Relaxed Movement**: Tension can hinder movement. Practitioners are encouraged to maintain a relaxed state, allowing for more natural and fluid motions during practice and combat.

3. Body Mechanics:

- **Joint Alignment**: Proper alignment of joints (e.g., knees, hips, shoulders) is critical for generating power and preventing injury. Practitioners learn to align their bodies correctly during techniques to maximize effectiveness.

- **Core Engagement**: Engaging the core muscles provides stability and strength, allowing for more powerful strikes and movements. A strong core facilitates better posture and balance.

4. Breath Coordination:

- **Synchronizing Breath and Movement**: Practitioners are taught to coordinate their breath with their movements, enhancing focus and power. For example, exhaling during a strike helps generate force, while inhaling can prepare for subsequent actions.

• **Mindful Awareness**: Breath awareness promotes mindfulness in movement, allowing practitioners to stay present and aware of their body dynamics throughout training.

5. Directional Movement:

• **Angle and Distance**: Understanding angles and distance is crucial for effective striking and defense. Practitioners learn to move in ways that optimize their position relative to opponents while maintaining effective range.

• **Circular Motion**: Many techniques in Haidong Gumdo utilize circular movements, enabling practitioners to generate power and momentum while maintaining fluidity.

6. Precision and Accuracy:

- **Targeting**: Precision in movement is essential for effective strikes. Practitioners are taught to focus on specific targets and ensure their techniques are directed accurately.

- **Controlled Execution**: Each movement should be executed with control and intention, enhancing both the effectiveness of the technique and the practitioner's ability to adapt to changing situations.

7. Adaptability:

- **Responsive Movement**: Practitioners must be able to adapt their movements based on the dynamics of sparring or self-defense situations. This involves recognizing opponents' movements and adjusting accordingly.

• **Situational Awareness**: Being aware of one's surroundings and adjusting movements based on environmental factors, such as space and potential obstacles, is vital for effective practice.

8. Practice of Techniques:

• **Repetition**: Mastery of movement principles comes through consistent practice of techniques, forms, and sparring. Repetition allows practitioners to internalize movements and develop muscle memory.

• **Feedback and Adjustment**: Practitioners are encouraged to seek feedback from instructors and peers, making necessary adjustments to their techniques and movements to improve performance.

The principles of movement in Haidong Gumdo are foundational to effective practice and mastery of the art. By focusing on balance, fluidity, body mechanics, breath coordination, and adaptability, practitioners can enhance their techniques, performance, and overall martial arts experience. Mastery of these principles not only improves physical skills but also fosters greater awareness and presence in both training and daily life.

The Mind-Body Connection

The mind-body connection is a vital concept in Haidong Gumdo that emphasizes the relationship between mental states and physical actions. This connection is integral to the practice, enhancing performance, focus, and overall well-being. Here are some key aspects of the mind-body connection in Haidong Gumdo:

1. Awareness and Presence:

• **Mindfulness in Movement**: Practitioners are encouraged to cultivate mindfulness, allowing them to be fully present during training. This heightened awareness helps improve focus and concentration, leading to more effective techniques.

• **Sensory Awareness**: Developing an acute awareness of physical sensations, such as balance, tension, and movement, enables practitioners to adjust their techniques and responses more effectively.

2. Mental Focus:

• **Concentration Techniques**: The ability to concentrate is crucial in martial arts. Practicing techniques with focused intent helps practitioners refine their skills and improve their performance.

- **Visualization**: Many practitioners use visualization techniques to mentally rehearse movements and strategies. This mental practice can enhance physical performance by reinforcing neural pathways associated with specific actions.

3. Emotional Regulation:

- **Managing Stress and Anxiety**: The mind-body connection allows practitioners to recognize and manage their emotional states. Techniques such as controlled breathing and meditation help reduce stress and anxiety, promoting emotional stability during training and competitions.

- **Building Confidence**: A strong mind-body connection fosters self-confidence and self-efficacy, allowing practitioners to approach challenges with a positive mindset.

4. Breath as a Bridge:

• **Breath Control**: Breath serves as a critical link between the mind and body. Practitioners learn to use breath control to regulate energy, maintain focus, and manage physical exertion.

• **Synchronizing Breath with Movement**: Coordinating breath with physical movements enhances the overall effectiveness of techniques, allowing for smoother transitions and greater power generation.

5. Holistic Development:

• **Integration of Mind and Body**: The practice of Haidong Gumdo emphasizes the integration of mental and physical training. Practitioners work on both technical skills and mental fortitude, recognizing that both aspects contribute to overall martial arts proficiency.

- **Personal Growth**: The mind-body connection facilitates personal growth, as practitioners learn to overcome mental barriers, cultivate resilience, and develop a deeper understanding of themselves through training.

6. Adaptability and Responsiveness:

- **Situational Awareness**: A strong mind-body connection enhances situational awareness, allowing practitioners to respond quickly and effectively to changing circumstances during sparring or self-defense scenarios.

- **Intuitive Movements**: Practitioners with a well-developed mind-body connection can execute techniques more intuitively, making split-second decisions based on their awareness of the environment and opponents.

7. Physical Conditioning:

• **Physical Fitness**: The mind-body connection emphasizes the importance of physical conditioning, helping practitioners understand how their physical state affects their mental clarity and focus.

• **Injury Prevention**: Being attuned to physical sensations allows practitioners to recognize potential injuries or strains early, helping them adjust their movements and reduce the risk of injury.

The mind-body connection is a foundational element of Haidong Gumdo that enhances both technical skills and personal growth. By cultivating awareness, focus, emotional regulation, and breath control, practitioners can develop a deeper understanding of themselves and their martial arts practice. This connection not only improves performance but also fosters overall well-being, making it an essential aspect of the Haidong Gumdo journey.

CHAPTER 2: TRAINING TECHNIQUES

Basic Cuts And Strikes

In Haidong Gumdo, mastering basic cuts and strikes is essential for developing effective swordsmanship and understanding the principles of movement. Here are some of the fundamental cuts and strikes commonly practiced:

1. Sang Gyeok (상격) - Upper Cut:

• **Description**: This cut is executed from a high position, striking downward toward an opponent's upper body or head.

• **Technique**: The sword is raised above the shoulder, and the cut is made in a diagonal or vertical motion, often finishing in a ready position.

2. Ara Gyeok (하격) - Lower Cut:

• **Description**: This cut is performed from a low position, aimed at the lower body or legs of the opponent.

• **Technique**: The sword starts at the hip and moves upward in a diagonal or vertical fashion, effectively targeting the opponent's lower areas.

3. Yup Gyeok (옆격) - Side Cut:

• **Description**: A horizontal cut that targets the opponent's side, often delivered from a lateral position.

• **Technique**: The sword is swung from one side to the other, utilizing hip rotation to generate power. This cut is essential for lateral attacks.

4. Gyeok Kkeut (격 끝) - End of Cut:

• **Description**: This refers to the finishing motion of a cut, ensuring that the blade comes to a complete stop in a controlled manner.

• **Technique**: After executing a cut, practitioners must practice proper follow-through and ensure the sword is positioned for defense or a subsequent attack.

5. Jeon Gyeok (전격) - Forward Cut:

• **Description**: This cut is delivered while advancing toward the opponent, typically aimed at the torso or head.

• **Technique**: Practitioners step forward while executing the cut, maintaining balance and control throughout the movement.

6. Dwi Gyeok (뒤격) - Back Cut:

• **Description**: A defensive cut executed while retreating or moving backward.

• **Technique**: This cut allows practitioners to maintain distance while countering an opponent's attack. The sword is moved backward in a controlled manner to deflect or strike.

7. Banjeong (반전) - Reverse Cut:

• **Description**: A cut performed in the opposite direction from a forward strike, often used to counter an incoming attack.

• **Technique**: Practitioners learn to pivot and redirect their movements, executing a cut that flows from the initial strike.

8. Dah (다) – Thrust:

• **Description**: This technique involves thrusting the sword directly at the opponent, targeting vulnerable areas such as the torso or face.

• **Technique**: The sword is thrust forward with both hands, using body weight and footwork to add power to the strike.

9. Bokkeum (복금) - Cut with Combination:

• **Description**: This refers to a series of cuts executed in quick succession to overwhelm an opponent.

• **Technique**: Practitioners practice combinations of upper, lower, and side cuts, emphasizing fluid transitions between each movement.

10. Sabeom Gyeok (사범격) - Instructor's Cut:

• **Description**: A fundamental cut taught by instructors, showcasing proper form and technique.

• **Technique**: This cut emphasizes precision and control, focusing on developing the practitioner's overall skills.

Mastering these basic cuts and strikes in Haidong Gumdo is essential for building a strong foundation in swordsmanship. Each cut has specific applications and techniques that contribute to a practitioner's overall skill set. Regular practice and refinement of these movements will lead to improved technique, power, and effectiveness in both training and sparring situations.

Footwork Fundamentals

Footwork is a crucial aspect of Haidong Gumdo, as it directly influences balance, mobility, and the effectiveness of techniques. Proper footwork allows practitioners to position themselves optimally for offense and defense. Here are the fundamental footwork principles and techniques practiced in Haidong Gumdo:

1. Basic Stance Transitions:

- **Joonbi Sogi (준비 자세) - Ready Stance**:

Practitioners begin in this position, with feet shoulder-width apart, ready to move into any technique.

- **Transitioning**: Smooth transitions between stances, such as from Joonbi Sogi to other stances, are essential for maintaining balance and readiness.

2. Stepping Techniques:

- **Chulgi (출기) - Forward Step**:
Practitioners step forward with one foot while maintaining balance and stability, often used to close the distance to an opponent.

- **Dwi Chulgi (뒤 출기) - Backward Step**:
This technique involves stepping back to create distance, allowing for defensive maneuvers or counterattacks.

- **Yup Chulgi (옆 출기) - Side Step**: A lateral movement to the left or right, helping practitioners evade attacks and reposition themselves for an effective strike.

3. Sliding Footwork:

• **Moori Chulgi (무리 출기) - Sliding Step**:

Practitioners slide their foot forward without lifting it entirely off the ground, maintaining a low center of gravity for stability.

• **Application**: This technique is useful for advancing toward an opponent while staying balanced and ready for immediate action.

4. Pivoting:

• **Bansan (반전) - Pivoting**: This involves turning on the balls of the feet to change direction quickly while maintaining balance.

• **Technique**: Practitioners learn to pivot effectively, allowing them to evade attacks or reposition for counterstrikes without losing balance.

5. Diagonal Movement:

- **Sang-Mool (상물) - Diagonal Step**: Stepping diagonally allows practitioners to approach opponents from different angles, making it harder for them to predict attacks.

- **Technique**: This movement helps in creating advantageous angles for strikes and defending against incoming attacks.

6. Combination Footwork:

- **Multiple Steps**: Practitioners combine different stepping techniques, such as stepping forward and then side-stepping, to create dynamic movement patterns during sparring or forms.

- **Fluid Transitions**: This enhances overall movement fluidity, allowing for quick adaptations during combat.

7. Balance and Stability:

- **Weight Distribution**: Practicing proper weight distribution between feet is vital for maintaining balance during movement. Practitioners learn to shift their weight appropriately to remain stable.

- **Core Engagement**: Engaging the core during footwork provides added stability and strength, allowing for more powerful strikes and defenses.

8. Foot Placement:

- **Foot Alignment**: Proper foot placement, including angles and distance from each other, is crucial for effective movement. Practitioners learn to position their feet to maximize mobility and balance.

- **Heel-to-Toe Alignment**: Maintaining a heel-to-toe alignment during movement helps improve balance and facilitates smoother transitions between stances.

9. Training Drills:

• **Shadow Practice**: Practicing footwork through shadow training, where practitioners simulate techniques without an opponent, helps refine movement and coordination.

• **Partner Drills**: Engaging in drills with partners allows practitioners to apply footwork in a dynamic environment, enhancing adaptability and responsiveness.

10. Integration with Techniques:

• **Combining Cuts and Footwork**: Practitioners learn to integrate footwork with cuts and strikes, ensuring that each movement is executed with precision and power.

• **Dynamic Sparring**: In sparring sessions, the combination of effective footwork and striking techniques allows practitioners to maintain an advantage over their opponents.

Mastering footwork fundamentals is essential for success in Haidong Gumdo. Proper footwork enhances balance, mobility, and the effectiveness of techniques, allowing practitioners to perform at their best in both training and sparring. By focusing on these principles and practicing regularly, practitioners can develop a solid foundation for their martial arts journey.

Sparring Techniques

Sparring in Haidong Gumdo is a critical component of training, providing practitioners with the opportunity to apply techniques in dynamic, real-time scenarios. Effective sparring requires a combination of technical skill, strategic thinking, and adaptability. Here are some fundamental sparring techniques and concepts practiced in Haidong Gumdo:

1. Defensive Techniques:

• **Blocking (막기)**: Practitioners learn various blocking techniques to defend against incoming strikes. Key blocks include:

• **Oren-Block (오렌 막기)**: A high block used to deflect upward strikes.

• **Dae-Block (대 막기)**: A low block aimed at stopping attacks targeting the lower body.

• **Evading (회피)**: Practitioners use footwork to evade attacks by stepping to the side or backward, creating distance from their opponents.

2. Counterattacks:

• **Immediate Response**: After successfully blocking or evading an attack, practitioners are trained to respond with a quick counterattack. This requires awareness and timing to capitalize on openings.

• **Combination Techniques**: Practitioners learn to follow up blocks with a series of strikes, integrating cuts and thrusts to create effective combinations.

3. Distance Management:

• **Controlling Distance**: Understanding how to control the distance between oneself and an opponent is vital in sparring. Practitioners learn when to close the distance for attacks and when to create space to avoid strikes.

• **Range Awareness**: Being aware of the effective range of both the sword and the opponent's movements helps practitioners make informed decisions during sparring.

4. Footwork in Sparring:

• **Dynamic Movement**: Effective footwork allows practitioners to change angles, evade strikes, and maintain balance while executing techniques. Practicing smooth transitions between steps is essential for effective sparring.

• **Positioning**: Proper positioning in relation to the opponent is key. Practitioners learn to use footwork to maintain advantageous angles for strikes while avoiding their opponent's line of attack.

5. Targeting:

• **Identifying Vulnerable Areas**: Practitioners are trained to target vulnerable areas on their opponents, such as the head, torso, and legs. Understanding where to strike effectively enhances the success of attacks.

• **Controlled Striking**: In sparring, practitioners focus on delivering strikes with control to avoid causing injury while still practicing realistic scenarios.

6. Strategy and Timing:

• **Reading Opponents**: Practitioners learn to read their opponent's movements and predict their actions, allowing for effective counters and strategic decisions.

• **Timing**: Developing a sense of timing is critical in sparring. Practitioners practice synchronizing their movements with their opponent's actions to maximize effectiveness.

7. Sparring Drills:

• **Controlled Sparring**: Practicing sparring with specific rules and limitations helps practitioners focus on particular techniques or strategies without overwhelming them.

• **Free Sparring**: Engaging in free sparring allows for the application of techniques in a more realistic and dynamic environment, fostering adaptability and creativity.

8. Mindset and Sportsmanship:

• **Mental Preparedness**: Sparring requires a calm and focused mindset. Practitioners are encouraged to stay relaxed and composed, allowing them to make better decisions during the exchange.

• **Respect and Sportsmanship**: Practicing good sportsmanship is essential. Practitioners learn to respect their opponents, instructors, and the art itself, fostering a positive training environment.

9. Situational Sparring:

• **Scenario Training**: Practicing specific scenarios or drills that mimic real-life situations helps practitioners develop skills for unexpected encounters.

• **Adapting to Different Styles**: Sparring with partners of varying skill levels and styles allows practitioners to adapt and learn from different techniques and approaches.

10. Post-Sparring Reflection:

• **Analyzing Performance**: After sparring sessions, practitioners are encouraged to reflect on their performance, identifying areas for improvement and successful techniques.

- **Feedback**: Receiving constructive feedback from instructors and peers helps practitioners refine their skills and enhance their overall performance.

Sparring techniques in Haidong Gumdo are essential for developing practical skills and enhancing overall martial arts proficiency. By focusing on defensive techniques, counterattacks, distance management, and strategic thinking, practitioners can improve their performance in sparring and gain valuable insights into their martial arts journey. Regular practice and reflection on sparring experiences will lead to continuous growth and improvement in Haidong Gumdo.

Forms (Hyung) And Their Significance

Forms, known as *Hyung* (형), are a fundamental aspect of Haidong Gumdo training. They consist of pre-arranged sequences of movements that simulate combat scenarios, allowing practitioners to practice techniques, improve their skills, and internalize the principles of the art. Here are key aspects of forms and their significance in Haidong Gumdo:

1. Understanding Forms (Hyung):

• **Definition**: Forms are structured patterns of movements that incorporate various techniques, including cuts, stances, and footwork. Each form consists of specific sequences that practitioners perform in a designated order.

• **Variations**: Different forms are designed for various skill levels, from beginner to advanced, allowing practitioners to progress through increasingly complex sequences.

2. Technique Refinement:

• **Precision and Accuracy**: Practicing forms helps practitioners refine their techniques, focusing on proper alignment, timing, and execution. Repetition of movements enhances muscle memory and promotes precision.

• **Control and Balance**: Forms require practitioners to maintain control over their movements and balance throughout the sequences. This focus on stability helps improve overall coordination and body mechanics.

3. Mental Discipline:

• **Focus and Concentration**: Executing forms demands a high level of concentration and mental engagement. Practitioners learn to focus their minds on the movements, enhancing their mental discipline and awareness.

• **Memory Development**: Learning and memorizing forms contribute to cognitive development, as practitioners must recall complex sequences of movements and apply them correctly.

4. Breath Control:

• **Synchronization**: Practitioners are taught to coordinate their breath with movements, enhancing the effectiveness of techniques and promoting relaxation. Controlled breathing helps maintain focus and energy during practice.

- **Energy Management**: Learning to manage breath during forms allows practitioners to sustain energy levels throughout the sequence, improving overall endurance.

5. Combat Simulation:

- **Application of Techniques**: Forms simulate combat scenarios, allowing practitioners to practice techniques in a controlled environment. This helps them understand how to apply skills during sparring or self-defense situations.

- **Strategic Thinking**: Practicing forms encourages practitioners to think strategically about their movements and techniques, developing an understanding of timing, distance, and angles.

6. Cultural and Historical Significance:

- **Tradition and Heritage**: Forms carry historical and cultural significance, connecting practitioners to the lineage of Haidong Gumdo and its martial arts traditions. This cultural awareness fosters a sense of respect and appreciation for the art.

- **Philosophical Foundations**: Many forms incorporate philosophical principles of martial arts, such as respect, humility, and perseverance. Practicing forms helps instill these values in practitioners.

7. Self-Expression and Creativity:

- **Personal Interpretation**: While forms are standardized, practitioners can express their individual style and interpretation during execution. This allows for creativity within the structured framework of forms.

• **Emotional Connection**: Practicing forms can evoke emotions and feelings, providing an opportunity for practitioners to connect with their martial arts journey on a deeper level.

8. Physical Conditioning:

• **Strength and Flexibility**: Regular practice of forms helps develop physical attributes, including strength, flexibility, and endurance. The movements engage various muscle groups, promoting overall fitness.

• **Cardiovascular Health**: Performing forms in a flowing manner contributes to cardiovascular health, as practitioners engage in continuous movement over extended periods.

9. Progress Tracking:

• **Skill Assessment**: Forms serve as a benchmark for evaluating progress in skill development. Instructors can assess a practitioner's mastery of techniques and overall proficiency through form performance.

• **Belt Promotion**: Mastery of specific forms is often a requirement for belt promotions, marking significant milestones in a practitioner's martial arts journey.

10. Integration with Sparring and Techniques:

• **Complementing Sparring**: Forms enhance sparring abilities by reinforcing techniques and movements practiced in a dynamic environment. They provide a foundation upon which sparring strategies can be built.

- **Holistic Training**: Practicing forms complements other training aspects, such as sparring, footwork, and meditation, contributing to a well-rounded martial arts education.

Forms (Hyung) in Haidong Gumdo are essential for developing technical skills, mental discipline, and physical conditioning. Through the practice of forms, practitioners refine their techniques, enhance focus, and connect with the rich traditions of martial arts. Mastering forms not only prepares practitioners for sparring and combat but also fosters personal growth, discipline, and self-expression within their martial arts journey.

Weapons Training Beyond The Sword

In Haidong Gumdo, while the sword is the primary focus, weapons training extends beyond it to encompass various traditional martial arts weapons. This training enriches practitioners' skills, enhances their understanding of weaponry, and contributes to their overall martial arts development. Here are some key aspects of weapons training beyond the sword in Haidong Gumdo:

1. Introduction to Additional Weapons

Bo Staff (봉):

• **Description**: A long wooden staff, typically around 6 feet in length, used for striking, blocking, and thrusting.

- **Training Focus**: Practitioners learn to utilize the staff for distance management, control, and versatility in both offense and defense.

Nunchaku (능착):

- **Description**: A traditional weapon consisting of two sticks connected by a chain or rope, used for striking and entangling.

- **Training Focus**: Practitioners develop coordination, agility, and precision, as well as enhance their reflexes through various techniques.

Sai (사이):

- **Description**: A three-pronged weapon with a long central blade and two shorter prongs, often used for thrusting and blocking.

• **Training Focus**: Practitioners focus on both offensive techniques and defensive maneuvers, including trapping and disarming.

Tonfa (돈파):

• **Description**: A weapon resembling a wooden baton with a handle, used for striking and blocking.

• **Training Focus**: Emphasis on rotational movements and angles, allowing practitioners to engage in close-quarters combat effectively.

2. Fundamentals of Weapon Handling:

• **Grip and Control**: Practicing proper grip techniques for each weapon to ensure control and maneuverability during use.

• **Balance and Stability**: Emphasizing body mechanics and posture to maintain balance while wielding various weapons.

3. Application of Techniques:

• **Translating Sword Techniques**: Many techniques learned with the sword can be adapted and applied to other weapons, helping practitioners understand the principles of weaponry.

• **Combining Techniques**: Practitioners learn to integrate strikes, blocks, and footwork from sword training into their weapons practice, creating a holistic approach to martial arts.

4. Defensive Strategies:

• **Blocking and Evasion**: Training includes defensive strategies specific to each weapon, teaching practitioners how to evade and counter attacks effectively.

• **Disarming Techniques**: Practitioners learn methods to disarm opponents using various weapons, emphasizing timing and precision.

5. Forms (Hyung) for Other Weapons:

• **Specific Forms**: Just as with the sword, forms are created for other weapons, allowing practitioners to practice sequences that enhance their understanding of movement and technique.

• **Progression through Forms**: Practicing forms helps practitioners build a repertoire of skills that can be applied in sparring or combat situations.

6. Sparring with Weapons:

- **Controlled Sparring**: Practicing sparring techniques with different weapons allows practitioners to apply their skills in a dynamic environment while maintaining safety.

- **Partner Drills**: Engaging in drills with partners helps practitioners develop timing, distance management, and adaptability when using weapons.

7. Historical and Cultural Context:

- **Understanding Weaponry**: Learning about the history and cultural significance of various weapons enhances practitioners' appreciation for martial arts traditions.

- **Martial Philosophy**: Exploring the philosophical principles behind weapons training fosters a deeper understanding of martial arts as a whole.

8. Physical Conditioning:

- **Strength and Endurance**: Training with various weapons helps develop overall physical fitness, including strength, coordination, and flexibility.

- **Dynamic Movement**: The diverse movements involved in weapons training promote cardiovascular health and agility.

9. Mindset and Discipline:

- **Focus and Concentration**: Weapons training requires a heightened level of focus and mental engagement, enhancing practitioners' overall mental discipline.

• **Respect for Weapons**: Emphasizing the importance of respect and responsibility when handling weapons is a key aspect of training, fostering a sense of humility and awareness.

10. Integration into Sparring and Forms:

• **Dynamic Practice**: Integrating weapons training into regular sparring sessions encourages practitioners to adapt and apply their skills in various contexts.

• **Holistic Development**: Training with multiple weapons contributes to a well-rounded martial arts education, allowing practitioners to explore different styles and techniques.

Weapons training beyond the sword in Haidong Gumdo enriches practitioners' skills and understanding of martial arts. By exploring various traditional weapons, practitioners develop versatility, coordination, and mental discipline. This training not only enhances their combat abilities but also deepens their appreciation for the history and philosophy of martial arts, contributing to a more comprehensive and fulfilling martial arts journey.

CHAPTER 3: ADVANCED TECHNIQUES

Mastering Advanced Cuts

Mastering advanced cuts in Haidong Gumdo is essential for developing a high level of proficiency in swordsmanship. Advanced cuts require precision, control, and an understanding of timing and distance. Here are key aspects of advanced cuts, including techniques, applications, and training methods:

1. Understanding Advanced Cuts: Advanced cuts are complex techniques that build on basic cuts, incorporating intricate movements, angles, and combinations to enhance effectiveness in combat.

• **Importance**: These cuts allow practitioners to engage with opponents more dynamically and create opportunities for follow-up attacks.

2. Key Advanced Cuts

Dah Gyeok (다 격) - Thrusting Cut:

• **Description**: A powerful thrust delivered at high speed, targeting vital areas such as the torso or neck.

• **Technique**: The practitioner steps forward while thrusting, maintaining a straight line from the sword to the target for maximum impact.

Hwa Gyeok (화격) - Flowing Cut:

• **Description**: A series of cuts performed in quick succession, creating a fluid and continuous motion that overwhelms the opponent.

• **Technique**: Practitioners learn to combine various cuts (e.g., upper, lower, and side) into a seamless flow, emphasizing timing and rhythm.

Sujeong Gyeok (수정격) - Refinement Cut:

• **Description**: A precise cut that targets an opponent's weapon to deflect or disarm them while simultaneously creating an opening for a follow-up strike.

• **Technique**: This cut requires an understanding of angles and timing, as practitioners must anticipate the opponent's movements.

Nae Gyeok (내격) - Inside Cut:

• **Description**: An inward cut aimed at the opponent's side or torso, often executed when the opponent is close.

• **Technique**: Practitioners learn to angle their cuts effectively to penetrate defenses and capitalize on openings.

Gyeok Tteul (격뜰) - Rising Cut:

• **Description**: A diagonal cut that rises from low to high, designed to target an opponent's upper body or head while simultaneously blocking low strikes.

• **Technique**: The cut is executed with a sweeping motion, incorporating body weight to generate power.

3. Applications of Advanced Cuts:

• **Offensive Strategy**: Advanced cuts are often used to initiate attacks or exploit openings in an opponent's defense, making them crucial for effective offensive strategies.

• **Defensive Techniques**: Many advanced cuts also serve a defensive purpose, allowing practitioners to block incoming strikes while simultaneously counterattacking.

4. Training Methods:

• **Repetition and Drills**: Practicing advanced cuts repeatedly helps refine technique and build muscle memory. Structured drills can focus on specific cuts or combinations.

• **Partner Work**: Sparring with partners allows practitioners to practice advanced cuts in dynamic scenarios, helping them understand timing and distance in real-time situations.

• **Forms (Hyung)**: Incorporating advanced cuts into forms provides an opportunity to practice them in a controlled environment while focusing on precision and fluidity.

5. Emphasis on Precision and Control:

• **Body Mechanics**: Practitioners must focus on proper body mechanics, including alignment and posture, to execute advanced cuts with precision and power.

• **Concentration**: Mastering advanced cuts requires intense concentration and awareness, ensuring that each movement is executed accurately and effectively.

6. Footwork Integration:

• **Dynamic Footwork**: Advanced cuts must be paired with effective footwork to enhance mobility and positioning. Practitioners learn to integrate foot movements that complement the cuts.

• **Creating Angles**: Effective footwork allows practitioners to create advantageous angles for their cuts, making them harder for opponents to defend against.

7. Timing and Distance Management:

• **Understanding Timing**: Practitioners learn to gauge the right moment to execute advanced cuts, allowing them to capitalize on openings while minimizing vulnerability.

• **Distance Control**: Mastery of distance is crucial; practitioners must be able to judge when to close the gap for an attack and when to maintain space for defense.

8. Mindset and Strategy:

• **Strategic Thinking**: Practicing advanced cuts encourages practitioners to think strategically, considering how to create openings and respond to opponents' actions.

• **Adaptability**: Mastering these techniques fosters adaptability, allowing practitioners to adjust their approach based on the dynamics of sparring or combat.

9. Feedback and Self-Reflection:

• **Instructor Feedback**: Regular feedback from instructors is essential for refining advanced cuts, as they can provide insights into technique and areas for improvement.

- **Self-Assessment**: Practitioners are encouraged to assess their own performance, reflecting on execution and making adjustments as needed.

10. Integration into Sparring:

- **Application in Sparring**: Practicing advanced cuts in sparring sessions allows practitioners to apply their techniques in a realistic setting, enhancing their combat effectiveness.

- **Combining Techniques**: Practitioners learn to combine advanced cuts with other techniques, such as blocks and counters, creating a more comprehensive skill set.

Mastering advanced cuts in Haidong Gumdo is essential for developing proficient swordsmanship and enhancing combat effectiveness. By focusing on precision, control, timing, and adaptability, practitioners can elevate their skills and deepen their understanding of the art.

Regular practice, feedback, and integration into sparring will lead to continuous improvement and mastery of advanced cuts, ultimately contributing to a more successful martial arts journey.

Defensive Techniques

Defensive techniques in Haidong Gumdo are essential for protecting oneself during combat while creating opportunities for counterattacks. These techniques help practitioners develop awareness, timing, and control in a variety of combat scenarios. Here are key aspects of defensive techniques, including specific methods and their significance:

1.   Fundamentals of Defensive Techniques:

• **Purpose**: The primary goal of defensive techniques is to minimize damage from an opponent's attack while creating openings for effective counterattacks.

• **Mindset**: Practitioners must maintain a calm and focused mindset to effectively anticipate and respond to incoming strikes.

2. Types of Defensive Techniques

A. Blocking Techniques:

- **High Block (오렌 막기)**: A technique used to deflect downward strikes aimed at the head or upper body.

- **Low Block (대 막기)**: This technique is aimed at deflecting attacks targeting the lower body, such as kicks or strikes aimed at the legs.

- **Side Block (옆 막기)**: A lateral block that helps protect against attacks coming from the side, often used against thrusts or strikes from an angle.

B. Evading Techniques:

- **Footwork and Movement**: Practitioners learn to use footwork to step back, pivot, or sidestep to avoid incoming attacks, maintaining balance while creating distance.

• **Body Angling**: Practicing the art of angling the body can help practitioners slip past strikes and create advantageous positions for counterattacks.

C. Parrying Techniques:

• **Deflection**: Utilizing the sword to deflect or redirect an opponent's attack rather than blocking it directly. This technique allows for a smoother transition into a counterattack.

• **Trapping**: Involves using the sword to trap the opponent's weapon momentarily, allowing for a quick follow-up strike.

D. Disarming Techniques:

• **Weapon Control**: Practitioners learn specific techniques to control or disarm an opponent's weapon through precise movements and leverage.

• **Counter-Disarming**: Techniques that enable a practitioner to counter an opponent's attempt to disarm them while maintaining control over their own weapon.

3. Situational Awareness:

• **Reading the Opponent**: Practicing the ability to read an opponent's movements, anticipating their attacks, and responding effectively with defensive techniques.

• **Environmental Awareness**: Understanding the surroundings can influence defensive strategies, allowing practitioners to use their environment to their advantage.

4. Integration with Offensive Techniques:

• **Counterattacks**: After successfully executing a defensive technique, practitioners should be prepared to follow up with a counterattack, utilizing openings created by their defensive actions.

• **Flowing Movements**: Practitioners learn to transition seamlessly from defense to offense, creating a fluid combat style.

5. Footwork and Movement:

• **Dynamic Movement**: Effective footwork is critical in defensive techniques, allowing practitioners to evade attacks while maintaining the ability to strike back.

- **Positioning**: Practitioners must focus on positioning to ensure they are in the best possible place to defend against and counteract an opponent's attack.

6. Breath Control:

- **Calming Breath**: Maintaining controlled breathing during defensive maneuvers can enhance focus and reduce stress, improving reaction times.

- **Energy Management**: Practicing breath control can help practitioners manage their energy levels throughout a combat scenario.

7. Mindset and Strategy:

- **Calmness Under Pressure**: Defensive techniques require practitioners to remain calm and composed, allowing for better decision-making in high-stress situations.

• **Tactical Thinking**: Understanding when to use each defensive technique strategically can significantly impact the effectiveness of a practitioner's overall combat strategy.

8. Training Methods:

• **Partner Drills**: Engaging in drills with partners helps practitioners practice defensive techniques in a dynamic environment, enhancing their responsiveness.

• **Controlled Sparring**: Practicing in controlled sparring scenarios enables practitioners to apply defensive techniques while adapting to various opponents' styles.

9. Feedback and Self-Assessment:

• **Instructor Guidance**: Receiving feedback from instructors on defensive techniques helps practitioners refine their skills and understand areas for improvement.

• **Self-Reflection**: Practitioners are encouraged to reflect on their defensive performance, identifying strengths and areas needing further practice.

10. Integration into Forms (Hyung):

• **Practice in Forms**: Many defensive techniques are incorporated into forms, allowing practitioners to practice them in a structured way while enhancing their overall skill set.

Defensive techniques in Haidong Gumdo are crucial for ensuring a practitioner's safety while creating opportunities for effective counterattacks. By mastering various blocking, evading, and disarming techniques, practitioners enhance their combat skills, develop situational awareness, and cultivate a strategic mindset.

Regular practice, coupled with feedback and self-reflection, will lead to continuous improvement and greater proficiency in defensive techniques, ultimately contributing to a successful martial arts journey.

Counter Techniques

Counter techniques in Haidong Gumdo are essential for responding to an opponent's attacks effectively and turning the tide of a confrontation. Mastering these techniques involves timing, precision, and an understanding of both offensive and defensive strategies. Here are key aspects of counter techniques, including specific methods, applications, and training tips:

1. Understanding Counter Techniques: Counter techniques are responses to an opponent's attack, allowing practitioners to exploit openings created by their opponent's actions.

• **Purpose**: The primary goal is to neutralize the opponent's attack while simultaneously launching an effective counterattack.

2. Types of Counter Techniques

A. Direct Counters:

• **Immediate Response**: Executing a technique directly in response to an opponent's attack, capitalizing on openings.

• **Example**: Performing a cut or thrust immediately after blocking an incoming strike, using the momentum to enhance the effectiveness of the counter.

B. Counter-Attack Techniques:

• **Combination of Defense and Offense**: Using defensive techniques (like a block or parry) to create an opening for a follow-up attack.

• **Example**: Blocking an overhead strike and transitioning into a diagonal cut to counterattack.

C. Redirection Techniques:

• **Deflecting the Attack**: Instead of blocking, practitioners can deflect or redirect an opponent's weapon, creating an opening for a counter.

• **Example**: A practitioner uses a side block to deflect an attack, then follows up with a thrust or slash.

D. Timing Counters:

• **Anticipation**: Practitioners learn to anticipate the opponent's actions, allowing them to respond with the appropriate technique just before the attack lands.

• **Example**: Executing a quick cut or thrust as the opponent commits to their attack.

E. Disarming Counters:

• **Weapon Control**: Techniques designed to disarm an opponent while countering their attack.

• **Example**: Using a twisting motion to redirect the opponent's weapon while simultaneously targeting their body.

3. Key Principles of Counter Techniques:

• **Timing**: Mastering the ability to recognize the right moment to counter is crucial. This requires a keen awareness of the opponent's movements and intentions.

• **Distance Management**: Practitioners must understand distance to effectively execute counters, ensuring they are close enough to strike while remaining out of reach of the opponent's attack.

• **Fluidity**: Counter techniques should flow seamlessly from defensive actions, allowing practitioners to transition smoothly between defense and offense.

4. Situational Awareness:

• **Reading the Opponent**: Practicing the ability to read an opponent's body language and movements, anticipating their attacks and planning counter techniques accordingly.

• **Environmental Awareness**: Understanding how the surroundings can influence counter strategies, allowing practitioners to use obstacles or terrain to their advantage.

5. Footwork and Movement:

• **Dynamic Footwork**: Effective counters often rely on good footwork, allowing practitioners to position themselves advantageously while executing techniques.

• **Angle Creation**: Moving at angles can help practitioners evade attacks and create openings for their counters.

6. Breath Control:

• **Calm and Focused**: Maintaining controlled breathing during combat can help practitioners stay calm and focused, allowing for better execution of counter techniques.

• **Energy Management**: Proper breath control helps manage energy levels, ensuring practitioners can maintain stamina throughout a sparring session.

7. Mindset and Strategy:

• **Composure Under Pressure**: Practicing counter techniques requires a calm and composed mindset, enabling practitioners to react effectively in high-stress situations.

• **Tactical Thinking**: Counter techniques encourage strategic thinking, allowing practitioners to consider various options and responses based on their opponent's actions.

8. Training Methods:

• **Partner Drills**: Engaging in drills with partners helps practitioners practice counter techniques in dynamic scenarios, enhancing their responsiveness.

• **Controlled Sparring**: Practicing counters in controlled sparring sessions allows practitioners to apply techniques in real-time and adapt to different opponents' styles.

9. Feedback and Self-Assessment:

• **Instructor Guidance**: Regular feedback from instructors on counter techniques helps practitioners refine their skills and understand areas for improvement.

• **Self-Reflection**: Practitioners are encouraged to assess their performance during sparring or drills, identifying successful counter techniques and areas that need further practice.

10. Integration into Forms (Hyung):

• **Practice in Forms**: Many counter techniques can be incorporated into forms, allowing practitioners to practice them in a structured manner while enhancing overall skill development.

Counter techniques in Haidong Gumdo are vital for effective combat and self-defense.

By mastering various direct counters, redirection techniques, and disarming methods, practitioners enhance their ability to respond to attacks and turn defensive situations into offensive opportunities.

Regular practice, combined with feedback and situational awareness, will lead to improved proficiency in counter techniques, ultimately contributing to a successful martial arts journey.

Combining Techniques For Self-Defense

Combining techniques for self-defense in Haidong Gumdo involves integrating various skills and strategies to create a cohesive response to an attack. This holistic approach enhances a practitioner's ability to adapt to dynamic situations, ensuring effectiveness in self-defense scenarios. Here are key aspects to consider when combining techniques for self-defense:

1.   Understanding   the   Self-Defense Context:

• **Real-Life Application**: Self-defense techniques should be practical and applicable in real-life situations. Practitioners must be able to assess threats and respond appropriately.

• **Legal Considerations**: Understanding the legal implications of self-defense in one's jurisdiction is crucial, as practitioners must know when and how to use force appropriately.

2. Key Techniques to Combine

A. Defensive Techniques:

- **Blocking**: Utilize blocking techniques to protect against incoming strikes.

- **Evading**: Incorporate footwork and body movement to evade attacks while positioning oneself for a counter.

B. Counter Techniques:

- **Immediate Counters**: After successfully blocking or evading, follow up with direct counterattacks such as cuts or thrusts.

- **Disarming**: Incorporate techniques to disarm an opponent while countering their attack, enhancing control over the situation.

C. Striking Techniques:

• **Combination Strikes**: Use a series of strikes, such as a combination of cuts and thrusts, to overwhelm an opponent.

• **Targeting Vulnerable Areas**: Focus on strikes aimed at vulnerable points on the opponent's body, such as the head, throat, or solar plexus.

3. Strategic Flow of Techniques:

• **Flowing Movement**: Techniques should flow seamlessly from one to another. For example, transitioning from a block to a counter, followed by a follow-up strike.

• **Rhythm and Timing**: Practitioners must develop a sense of rhythm and timing to ensure that their movements are coordinated and effective.

4. Footwork Integration:

• **Dynamic Footwork**: Use footwork to create angles and maintain distance, allowing for effective defense and counterattacks.

• **Positioning**: Good positioning is critical for executing techniques effectively and maintaining control over the encounter.

5. Breath Control and Focus:

• **Controlled Breathing**: Maintaining calm and controlled breathing during self-defense scenarios enhances focus and reduces stress, enabling clearer decision-making.

• **Mental Focus**: Practitioners must cultivate mental focus to remain aware of their surroundings and respond appropriately to threats.

6. Mindset and Awareness:

• **Situational Awareness**: Being aware of one's surroundings and potential threats is crucial for effective self-defense. Practitioners should constantly assess their environment.

• **Composure Under Pressure**: Remaining calm in high-stress situations allows for better execution of combined techniques.

7. Practical Training Methods:

• **Scenario-Based Training**: Engage in scenario-based drills that simulate real-life self-defense situations. This helps practitioners practice combining techniques under pressure.

• **Partner Drills**: Work with partners to practice defensive and counter techniques, focusing on timing and responsiveness in dynamic environments.

8. Feedback and Improvement:

• **Instructor Guidance**: Regular feedback from instructors helps practitioners refine their technique combinations, improving overall effectiveness.

• **Self-Assessment**: Encourage practitioners to reflect on their performance during drills and sparring, identifying strengths and areas for improvement.

9. Integration into Forms (Hyung):

• **Practice in Forms**: Incorporate self-defense techniques into forms to reinforce muscle memory and fluidity in movements, allowing for more instinctive responses during actual encounters.

Combining techniques for self-defense in Haidong Gumdo is essential for creating effective responses to various threats. By integrating defensive techniques, counterattacks, and striking methods, practitioners can develop a well-rounded self-defense strategy. Continuous practice, situational awareness, and the ability to remain calm under pressure will enhance proficiency and confidence, contributing to a successful martial arts journey.

Using Environment And Adaptability

Using the environment and adaptability in Haidong Gumdo is crucial for enhancing a practitioner's effectiveness in self-defense and combat situations. Understanding how to leverage one's surroundings and adapt to changing circumstances can significantly improve a martial artist's performance. Here are key aspects to consider:

1. Environmental Awareness:

• **Assessing Surroundings**: Practitioners must develop the ability to quickly assess their environment for potential hazards or advantages. This includes identifying obstacles, escape routes, and objects that can be used for defense or offense.

• **Utilizing Terrain**: Understanding the terrain can impact movement and strategy. For example, practicing on uneven surfaces or inclines can help practitioners learn to maintain balance and adapt their techniques.

2. Adapting Techniques to the Environment:

• **Spatial Awareness**: Practitioners should be aware of the space around them and adjust their techniques accordingly. In a confined space, techniques may need to be modified for effective execution.

• **Using Objects**: The environment may contain objects that can be utilized in combat, such as walls for support, furniture for obstacles, or items that can be used as improvised weapons (e.g., sticks, chairs).

3. Adapting Footwork and Movement:

• **Dynamic Footwork**: Practitioners must adapt their footwork to navigate different surfaces (e.g., slippery floors, uneven ground) while maintaining balance and control.

• **Positioning**: Utilizing the environment to position oneself advantageously can help in both offense and defense. For example, backing an opponent against a wall limits their movement options.

4.   Responding   to   Unpredictable Situations:

• **Improvisation**: The ability to think on one's feet and improvise techniques based on the unfolding situation is vital. Practitioners should practice scenarios where they need to adapt their techniques quickly.

• **Scenario Training**: Engage in drills that simulate unexpected changes in the environment, such as sudden obstacles or multiple attackers, to develop adaptability and quick decision-making skills.

5. Mental Adaptability:

• **Flexible Mindset**: Cultivating a flexible mindset enables practitioners to adjust their strategies and techniques based on the situation at hand. This includes being open to modifying techniques that may not be working as expected.

• **Problem-Solving**: Practitioners should focus on developing problem-solving skills, allowing them to identify effective responses in the heat of the moment.

6. Integrating Environmental Elements into Training:

• **Obstacle Courses**: Create training scenarios that incorporate obstacles, requiring practitioners to navigate while executing techniques.

• **Natural Settings**: Practice techniques in outdoor environments to enhance adaptability to different surfaces, conditions, and situations.

7. Practical Application of Environment and Adaptability:

- **Combining Techniques with Environmental Awareness**: Encourage practitioners to think about how they can combine techniques with their understanding of the environment. For example, using a low block to redirect an attack into a wall or another object.

- **Use of Cover**: Teach practitioners to use cover (e.g., walls, vehicles) effectively during self-defense situations, allowing them to protect themselves while preparing for a counterattack.

8. Situational Training:

- **Role-Playing Scenarios**: Engage in role-playing exercises that simulate real-world situations, allowing practitioners to practice adapting their techniques in various environments.

• **Partner Drills**: Work with partners to create unpredictable scenarios where one practitioner attacks, and the other must adapt their response using environmental elements.

9. Feedback and Improvement:

• **Instructor Insights**: Encourage instructors to provide feedback on how effectively practitioners utilize their environment during training and combat.

• **Self-Assessment**: Practitioners should regularly assess their performance and adaptability in different environments, identifying areas for improvement.

10. Developing Intuition:

• **Instinctive Responses**: Over time, practitioners can develop an intuitive understanding of how to adapt techniques based on their surroundings. This comes with experience and practice.

• **Situational Awareness Drills**: Engage in drills that enhance situational awareness, helping practitioners recognize when and how to utilize their environment effectively.

Using the environment and adaptability in Haidong Gumdo enhances a practitioner's self-defense capabilities and overall effectiveness in combat. By developing environmental awareness, adapting techniques to fit different situations, and fostering a flexible mindset, practitioners can become more versatile martial artists.

Regular practice, scenario training, and continuous self-reflection will contribute to greater proficiency and confidence in utilizing the environment to one's advantage.

CHAPTER 4: APPLICATION AND STRATEGY

Application In Real-Life Scenarios

The application of Haidong Gumdo techniques in real-life scenarios is crucial for practitioners to effectively use their skills in self-defense and combat situations. Understanding how to translate training into practical responses can make a significant difference in the outcome of an encounter. Here are key aspects to consider when applying Haidong Gumdo in real-life situations:

1. Situational Awareness:

• **Observation**: Practitioners should develop the habit of observing their surroundings and identifying potential threats. This includes being aware of people, objects, and exit routes.

- **Reading Body Language**: Recognizing changes in an opponent's body language can provide insight into their intentions, allowing practitioners to anticipate attacks.

2. Assessing Threat Levels:

- **Identifying Risks**: Understanding the difference between low and high-risk situations helps practitioners determine whether to engage or retreat.

- **De-escalation Techniques**: Practitioners should be equipped with skills to de-escalate tense situations verbally before they escalate to physical confrontation.

3. Applying Defensive Techniques:

- **Blocking and Evasion**: Using blocking techniques to defend against strikes while employing footwork to evade attacks can be essential in protecting oneself.

- **Creating Distance**: Maintaining a safe distance from an aggressor can provide time to assess the situation and decide on the appropriate response.

4. Utilizing Counter Techniques:

- **Immediate Counters**: After defending against an attack, practitioners can quickly launch counterattacks to neutralize the threat, utilizing techniques such as cuts, thrusts, or strikes to vulnerable areas.

- **Flowing Transitions**: Practicing the transition from defense to offense can enhance a practitioner's ability to respond fluidly in a real confrontation.

5. Environmental Utilization:

- **Using Surroundings**: Practitioners should learn to use their environment to their advantage, such as positioning themselves near walls, obstacles, or using objects as improvised weapons.

•   **Adaptive Strategies**: Practicing techniques that account for different environments (e.g., tight spaces, uneven terrain) can enhance adaptability in real situations.

6. Combining Techniques for Effectiveness:

• **Technique Combinations**: Practitioners can combine defensive and offensive techniques to create effective responses, such as blocking an attack followed by a swift counter.

•   **Flowing Movements**: Emphasizing fluidity between techniques can increase effectiveness during an encounter, allowing for quick adaptations based on the opponent's actions.

7. Mental Preparedness:

• **Calmness Under Pressure**: Developing a calm and focused mindset allows practitioners to think clearly during stressful situations, improving decision-making.

• **Visualization Techniques**: Practicing mental imagery and visualization can prepare practitioners for potential encounters, enhancing their confidence and readiness.

8. Scenario-Based Training:

• **Realistic Drills**: Engaging in scenario-based training that mimics real-life situations can help practitioners practice applying techniques under realistic conditions.

• **Role-Playing Exercises**: Practicing with partners in role-playing scenarios can help practitioners develop their responses to various threats and challenges.

9. Legal and Ethical Considerations:

- **Understanding Self-Defense Laws**: Practitioners should be aware of the legal implications of using martial arts techniques in self-defense situations, including when it is justified to engage physically.

- **Ethical Decision-Making**: Knowing when to disengage or use physical force is crucial for responsible martial arts practice.

10. Continuous Improvement:

- **Reflecting on Experiences**: After real-life encounters or training scenarios, practitioners should reflect on their performance and identify areas for improvement.

- **Feedback from Instructors**: Regular feedback from instructors can help practitioners refine their techniques and strategies for real-life applications.

The application of Haidong Gumdo techniques in real-life scenarios requires a combination of situational awareness, mental preparedness, and practical skill execution. By understanding how to assess threats, utilize defensive and counter techniques, and adapt to their environment, practitioners can enhance their effectiveness in self-defense situations. Continuous practice, scenario training, and reflection will contribute to greater proficiency and confidence in applying Haidong Gumdo in real-life encounters.

CHAPTER 5: THE ROLE OF SPARRING

Types Of Sparring

Sparring in Haidong Gumdo is an essential aspect of training, allowing practitioners to apply their techniques in dynamic, controlled environments. Different types of sparring serve various purposes, from skill development to preparation for real-life situations. Here are the primary types of sparring practiced in Haidong Gumdo:

1. Drill Sparring:

• **Purpose**: To practice specific techniques in a controlled environment.

• **Description**: Partners take turns executing pre-determined techniques or combinations, focusing on accuracy and control rather than full power. This type of sparring helps refine techniques and builds confidence.

• **Example**: One practitioner attacks with a specific strike while the other defends using a particular technique, then they switch roles.

2. Controlled Sparring:

• **Purpose**: To simulate combat scenarios while minimizing risk.

• **Description**: Practitioners engage in sparring with limited intensity and contact. They may wear protective gear and agree on rules to ensure safety. This type of sparring allows for the exploration of timing, distance, and technique application.

• **Example**: Practitioners spar with specific limitations, such as only targeting certain areas of the body or only using particular techniques.

3. Full-Contact Sparring:

• **Purpose**: To experience realistic combat situations and improve reflexes.

• **Description**: Practitioners engage in sparring with full power and intensity, using appropriate protective gear. This type of sparring mimics actual combat scenarios and helps develop resilience, reaction times, and the ability to apply techniques under pressure.

• **Example**: Practitioners spar freely, using all techniques within the guidelines of the dojo, focusing on realistic application.

4. One-on-Multiple Sparring:

• **Purpose**: To develop adaptability and decision-making under pressure.

• **Description**: A single practitioner faces multiple opponents in a sparring session. This type of sparring enhances situational awareness, movement, and the ability to manage multiple threats simultaneously.

• **Example**: One practitioner defends against attacks from two or more partners, practicing evasive maneuvers and counter techniques.

5. Scenario Sparring:

• **Purpose**: To prepare practitioners for real-life situations.

• **Description**: Practitioners engage in sparring that simulates specific scenarios, such as defending against an ambush, dealing with a weapon, or escaping from a hold. This type of sparring focuses on applying techniques in practical situations.

- **Example**: Practitioners may simulate being cornered or attacked unexpectedly and must respond using their skills.

6. Technical Sparring:

- **Purpose**: To focus on refining specific techniques or combinations.

- **Description**: Practitioners spar with a specific goal in mind, such as practicing footwork, counters, or weapon techniques. This type of sparring emphasizes skill refinement over competition.

- **Example**: A session dedicated to practicing various cuts and strikes while maintaining proper form and technique.

7. Conditioning Sparring:

- **Purpose**: To build endurance and physical fitness.

• **Description**: Practitioners engage in light sparring for extended periods, focusing on movement and maintaining energy levels rather than intensity. This type of sparring enhances stamina and builds the ability to maintain composure during prolonged encounters.

• **Example**: Practitioners spar for several minutes at a lower intensity, working on movement, breath control, and technique.

8. Free Sparring:

• **Purpose**: To encourage creativity and adaptability in techniques.

• **Description**: Practitioners spar without restrictions on techniques or targets, allowing them to experiment and apply what they've learned. This type of sparring fosters innovation and personal style.

• **Example**: Practitioners engage in open sparring sessions, applying various techniques and strategies spontaneously.

9. Cooperative Sparring:

• **Purpose**: To practice techniques and improve understanding between partners.

• **Description**: Practitioners work together to help each other learn and refine techniques, focusing on timing, positioning, and execution without the pressure of competition. This type of sparring emphasizes communication and partnership.

• **Example**: Practitioners may agree to alternate roles, with one attacking and the other defending, providing feedback on each other's techniques.

Understanding the various types of sparring in Haidong Gumdo is essential for developing a well-rounded skill set. Each type serves a unique purpose, from refining techniques to simulating real-life scenarios.

By engaging in different sparring methods, practitioners can enhance their abilities, build confidence, and prepare for various situations, ultimately contributing to their growth as martial artists. Regular practice of these sparring types can lead to improved reflexes, adaptability, and proficiency in Haidong Gumdo techniques.

Analysis Of Sparring Techniques

Analyzing sparring techniques in Haidong Gumdo is essential for understanding their effectiveness, applicability, and areas for improvement. This analysis encompasses various aspects of sparring, including technique execution, timing, distance management, and adaptability. Here's a comprehensive breakdown of key elements to consider when analyzing sparring techniques:

1. Technique Execution:

• **Precision and Accuracy**: Assess how accurately techniques are executed during sparring. Are the cuts, strikes, and blocks hitting their intended targets? Precision is vital in ensuring effectiveness during an encounter.

• **Form and Posture**: Analyze the practitioner's stance, grip, and overall body posture. Proper form contributes to the strength and effectiveness of techniques. Look for alignment and stability during movement.

• **Fluidity of Movement**: Evaluate the smoothness of transitions between techniques. Practitioners should move seamlessly from one technique to another without hesitation, demonstrating fluidity and control.

2. Timing:

• **Anticipation**: Analyze the practitioner's ability to anticipate an opponent's movements. Effective sparring involves recognizing cues that indicate an opponent's actions and responding appropriately.

• **Speed of Execution**: Evaluate how quickly techniques are executed in response to an opponent's actions. Quick reflexes are essential for effective sparring, allowing practitioners to capitalize on openings.

• **Timing of Attacks and Counters**: Examine the timing of both offensive and defensive techniques. Practitioners should recognize when to strike and when to defend, ensuring they act at the right moment.

3. Distance Management:

• **Proximity to Opponent**: Assess how well practitioners manage distance during sparring. Proper distance allows for effective striking while minimizing the risk of being hit.

• **Footwork**: Analyze the use of footwork for positioning and distance control. Practitioners should use footwork to create angles, evade attacks, and maintain an advantageous position.

• **Adjustments to Distance**: Evaluate the ability to adjust distance in response to an opponent's movements. Practitioners should be able to close the distance for an attack or create space for defense as needed.

4. Defensive Techniques:

• **Blocking and Evasion**: Analyze the effectiveness of defensive techniques. Are practitioners successfully blocking or evading attacks? This includes assessing their ability to read an opponent's movements and respond appropriately.

• **Counterattacks**: Evaluate the ability to execute counterattacks immediately after a defensive maneuver. Practitioners should strive to capitalize on openings created by an opponent's attacks.

5. Adaptability:

• **Responding to Unpredictability**: Assess how well practitioners adapt to unexpected moves from their opponents. This includes improvising techniques or switching strategies based on changing circumstances.

- **Environmental Adaptation**: Evaluate the ability to adapt techniques based on the sparring environment, whether it's a dojo, an outdoor setting, or a confined space.

6. Strategic Thinking:

- **Game Plan**: Analyze whether practitioners have a strategic approach to sparring. This includes having a plan for how to approach an opponent and adjusting tactics based on their actions.

- **Reading Opponents**: Evaluate the ability to read an opponent's strategies and adapt accordingly. This includes recognizing patterns and making tactical adjustments.

7. Mental Focus:

• **Calmness Under Pressure**: Analyze how well practitioners maintain composure during sparring. Mental clarity is crucial for effective decision-making and technique execution.

• **Confidence**: Assess the level of confidence displayed during sparring. Confidence can affect performance, influencing how techniques are executed and risks taken.

8. Feedback and Self-Reflection:

• **Instructor and Peer Feedback**: Encourage practitioners to seek feedback from instructors and peers regarding their performance. Constructive criticism can provide insights into areas for improvement.

- **Self-Assessment**: Practitioners should reflect on their sparring experiences, identifying strengths and weaknesses in their technique execution and overall performance.

9. Integration of Techniques:

- **Combining Techniques**: Evaluate the ability to integrate different techniques seamlessly during sparring. Practitioners should be able to flow between defensive and offensive moves effectively.

- **Use of Sets and Combinations**: Analyze the use of sets and combinations in sparring. Practitioners should utilize specific sequences of techniques that flow together naturally.

10. Physical Conditioning:

• **Stamina and Endurance**: Assess the physical condition of practitioners during sparring sessions. Good conditioning allows for sustained performance throughout the sparring session.

• **Strength and Agility**: Evaluate the strength and agility displayed during sparring. Practitioners should demonstrate the ability to generate power in their strikes and move quickly.

Analyzing sparring techniques in Haidong Gumdo provides valuable insights into practitioners' skills and areas for improvement. By focusing on technique execution, timing, distance management, adaptability, and mental focus, practitioners can enhance their sparring effectiveness. Continuous self-assessment and feedback from instructors and peers will contribute to ongoing development and proficiency in Haidong Gumdo. Regular analysis of sparring techniques not only improves performance but also prepares practitioners for real-life scenarios, ensuring they can effectively apply their skills when needed.

CHAPTER 6: HEALTH AND WELLNESS
Physical Conditioning And Training Regimen

Physical conditioning and a structured training regimen are crucial for practitioners of Haidong Gumdo, as they enhance strength, flexibility, endurance, and overall martial arts performance. Here's a comprehensive guide on physical conditioning and an effective training regimen for Haidong Gumdo practitioners:

1. Goals of Physical Conditioning:

• **Strength Development**: Build muscular strength to enhance the power of strikes and overall physical capabilities.

• **Endurance**: Improve cardiovascular endurance to sustain performance during sparring and long training sessions.

• **Flexibility**: Increase flexibility to execute techniques with a full range of motion and reduce the risk of injury.

• **Balance and Coordination**: Enhance balance and coordination for better movement control during techniques and sparring.

2. Components of a Conditioning Program

A. Strength Training:

• **Weight Training**: Incorporate compound movements such as squats, deadlifts, bench presses, and rows to build overall strength. Focus on lower and upper body strength as well as core stability.

• **Bodyweight Exercises**: Include push-ups, pull-ups, lunges, and planks to develop functional strength that translates to martial arts movements.

• **Resistance Bands**: Use resistance bands for exercises targeting specific muscle groups, enhancing strength and flexibility.

B. Cardiovascular Conditioning:

• **Aerobic Training**: Engage in activities such as running, cycling, swimming, or rowing to improve cardiovascular endurance. Aim for at least 20-30 minutes of moderate to vigorous aerobic exercise, 3-5 times per week.

• **High-Intensity Interval Training (HIIT)**: Incorporate HIIT workouts to improve cardiovascular fitness and stamina. Alternate between short bursts of intense activity (e.g., sprints or jumping jacks) and rest periods.

• **Circuit Training**: Create circuits combining strength and cardio exercises, allowing for varied training that builds endurance while developing strength.

C. Flexibility Training:

• **Dynamic Stretching**: Incorporate dynamic stretches before workouts to warm up muscles and prepare them for activity. Focus on movements that mimic martial arts techniques.

• **Static Stretching**: After workouts, perform static stretches to improve flexibility and prevent muscle tightness. Target major muscle groups used in Haidong Gumdo, such as the hamstrings, quadriceps, hips, and shoulders.

• **Yoga or Pilates**: Consider integrating yoga or Pilates into the training regimen to enhance flexibility, balance, and core strength.

D. Balance and Coordination:

• **Balance Exercises**: Include exercises such as single-leg stands, balance board workouts, or stability ball exercises to enhance balance and core stability.

• **Agility Drills**: Practice agility drills such as ladder drills or cone drills to improve footwork and coordination, essential for effective sparring and movement.

3. Training Regimen Structure

A. Weekly Training Plan:

Monday:

• Strength Training (Upper Body Focus)

• Flexibility Training

Tuesday:

• Sparring Drills

• Cardiovascular Conditioning (HIIT)

Wednesday:

• Strength Training (Lower Body Focus)

• Balance and Coordination Exercises

Thursday:

• Forms (Hyung) Practice

• Flexibility Training

Friday:

• Sparring Techniques and Drills

• Cardiovascular Conditioning (Steady-State)

Saturday:

• Full-Body Strength Training

• Agility Drills

Sunday:

• Rest and Recovery (light stretching or yoga)

B. Daily Warm-Up and Cool Down:

• **Warm-Up**: Begin each training session with a 10-15 minute warm-up, including dynamic stretches and light cardio to increase heart rate and prepare muscles.

• **Cool Down**: End each session with a 5-10 minute cool down that includes static stretching to improve flexibility and aid recovery.

4. Recovery and Nutrition:

• **Hydration**: Ensure adequate hydration before, during, and after training to maintain performance levels and promote recovery.

• **Nutrition**: Follow a balanced diet rich in lean proteins, complex carbohydrates, healthy fats, and a variety of fruits and vegetables. Proper nutrition supports energy levels, muscle recovery, and overall health.

• **Rest and Recovery**: Prioritize rest days to allow muscles to recover. Incorporate activities like foam rolling, massages, or light yoga to aid recovery.

5. Tracking Progress:

• **Set Goals**: Establish short-term and long-term goals related to strength, endurance, flexibility, and technique proficiency.

- **Monitor Performance**: Keep track of workout routines, progress, and achievements. Adjust the training regimen based on performance and personal goals.

A comprehensive physical conditioning and training regimen is essential for Haidong Gumdo practitioners to improve their performance, endurance, and overall effectiveness in martial arts. By focusing on strength, cardiovascular fitness, flexibility, balance, and coordination, practitioners can enhance their skills and prepare for the demands of sparring and real-life applications. Regular assessment and adjustment of the training regimen will ensure continuous improvement and growth as martial artists.

Nutrition For Martial Artists

Nutrition plays a vital role in the performance, recovery, and overall health of martial artists, including practitioners of Haidong Gumdo. A well-balanced diet can enhance physical conditioning, increase energy levels, and improve focus during training and competitions. Here's a comprehensive guide on nutrition tailored for martial artists:

1. Nutritional Goals for Martial Artists:

• **Enhance Performance**: Provide energy and nutrients to support training, sparring, and competition.

• **Facilitate Recovery**: Promote muscle repair and recovery after intense training sessions.

• **Maintain Optimal Weight**: Support body composition goals, whether for weight loss, maintenance, or muscle gain.

• **Boost Immune Function**: Strengthen the immune system to reduce the risk of illness and injury.

2. Macronutrient Breakdown: A balanced diet for martial artists should include appropriate proportions of macronutrients: carbohydrates, proteins, and fats.

A. Carbohydrates (50-60% of daily intake):

• **Role**: The primary source of energy for physical activities, especially high-intensity training and sparring.

Sources:

• **Complex Carbohydrates**: Whole grains (brown rice, quinoa, oats), starchy vegetables (sweet potatoes, corn), legumes (beans, lentils), and fruits.

• **Simple Carbohydrates**: Natural sugars found in fruits and dairy; use sparingly for quick energy.

B. Proteins (15-25% of daily intake):

• **Role**: Essential for muscle repair, recovery, and growth. Important for maintaining lean muscle mass.

Sources:

• **Lean Proteins**: Chicken, turkey, fish, eggs, tofu, tempeh, and low-fat dairy products.

• **Plant-Based Proteins**: Lentils, chickpeas, quinoa, nuts, and seeds.

C. Fats (20-30% of daily intake):

• **Role**: Provide essential fatty acids, support cell function, and help with hormone production.

Sources:

• **Healthy Fats**: Avocados, nuts, seeds, olive oil, coconut oil, and fatty fish (salmon, mackerel).

3. Micronutrients:

• Vitamins and minerals are crucial for overall health and performance. Focus on a varied diet rich in fruits and vegetables to ensure adequate intake of essential micronutrients.

• **Vitamin C**: Supports immune function and aids in recovery. Found in citrus fruits, bell peppers, strawberries, and broccoli.

• **Vitamin D**: Important for bone health and immune function. Sources include sunlight, fatty fish, fortified dairy, and egg yolks.

• **Calcium**: Essential for bone health. Found in dairy products, leafy greens, and fortified plant-based milk.

• **Iron**: Vital for oxygen transport in the blood. Sources include red meat, poultry, fish, lentils, and spinach.

4. Hydration:

• **Importance**: Adequate hydration is crucial for maintaining performance, regulating body temperature, and preventing dehydration.

Recommendations:

• Drink water before, during, and after training sessions.

• Consider electrolyte-replenishing drinks during intense or prolonged workouts.

• Monitor hydration levels by checking urine color; pale yellow indicates good hydration.

5. Meal Timing and Frequency:

• **Pre-Training Meals**: Consume a balanced meal containing carbohydrates and protein 2-3 hours before training. This can provide sustained energy.

• **Example**: Whole grain toast with nut butter and banana, or chicken with brown rice and vegetables.

- **Post-Training Recovery**: Focus on refueling with carbohydrates and protein within 30-60 minutes after training to aid recovery.

- **Example**: A protein shake with a banana, or a meal with lean protein and whole grains (grilled chicken and quinoa salad).

- **Snacks**: Include healthy snacks throughout the day to maintain energy levels and avoid fatigue.

- **Examples**: Greek yogurt with berries, apple slices with almond butter, or hummus with carrot sticks.

6. Supplements: While it's best to obtain nutrients from whole foods, some martial artists may benefit from supplements:

- **Protein Powder**: Useful for meeting protein needs, especially post-workout.

• **Creatine**: Can enhance strength and performance in high-intensity training.

• **Multivitamins**: May help fill nutrient gaps if dietary intake is insufficient.

7. Special Considerations:

• **Weight Management**: For practitioners needing to lose or gain weight, focus on gradual changes in diet and physical activity. Consult a nutritionist for personalized guidance.

• **Food Sensitivities and Allergies**: Tailor the diet to accommodate any food allergies or sensitivities to maintain health and performance.

Nutrition is a cornerstone of success for martial artists in Haidong Gumdo. By focusing on a balanced intake of macronutrients, micronutrients, and proper hydration, practitioners can enhance their performance, support recovery, and maintain overall health. A well-structured nutrition plan, tailored to individual needs and goals, will contribute significantly to their effectiveness and longevity in martial arts training.

Injury Prevention And Recovery

Injury prevention and recovery are critical components of training for martial artists, including practitioners of Haidong Gumdo. Effective strategies can help minimize the risk of injuries and facilitate faster recovery when they occur. Here's a comprehensive guide to injury prevention and recovery for martial artists:

1. Injury Prevention Strategies

A. Proper Warm-Up and Cool Down:

• **Warm-Up**: Always start with a dynamic warm-up before training to increase blood flow, enhance flexibility, and prepare muscles for activity. This may include:

1. Light cardio (jogging, jumping jacks)
2. Dynamic stretches (leg swings, arm circles)
3. Sport-specific movements (shadow fighting, footwork drills)

• **Cool Down**: After training, perform a cool-down routine that includes static stretching to improve flexibility and aid recovery.

B. Strength and Conditioning:

• **Muscle Balance**: Focus on strengthening both agonist (primary movers) and antagonist (opposing) muscle groups to maintain balance and reduce the risk of strains and imbalances.

• **Core Strength**: Develop core strength through targeted exercises (planks, Russian twists) to support overall stability and prevent injuries, especially in dynamic movements.

C. Flexibility Training:

• **Regular Stretching**: Incorporate flexibility training into your routine. Stretching helps maintain a full range of motion and prevents tightness that can lead to injury.

• **Yoga or Pilates**: Consider practicing yoga or Pilates to enhance flexibility, balance, and body awareness.

D. Technique Mastery:

• **Focus on Fundamentals**: Prioritize mastering proper techniques in stances, strikes, and footwork to reduce the risk of injuries caused by improper form.

• **Seek Instruction**: Regularly seek feedback from instructors to ensure techniques are executed safely and correctly.

E. Gradual Progression:

• **Increase Intensity Gradually**: Avoid sudden increases in training intensity or volume. Gradually build up the difficulty of workouts to prevent overuse injuries.

• **Cross-Training**: Incorporate different training modalities to avoid repetitive strain on specific muscle groups and joints.

F. Rest and Recovery:

• **Adequate Rest**: Ensure adequate rest and recovery between training sessions to allow muscles and joints to heal and adapt.

• **Listen to Your Body**: Pay attention to signs of fatigue or discomfort. Take breaks as needed and avoid pushing through pain.

2. Common Martial Arts Injuries: Understanding common injuries can help practitioners be more vigilant in prevention efforts.

• **Sprains and Strains**: Typically occur in the ankle, knee, or wrist due to improper landing, twisting, or overextension.

- **Contusions**: Bruises from strikes or impacts during sparring or training.

- **Fractures**: Occur due to high-impact collisions or falls.

- **Tendonitis**: Inflammation of tendons, often due to repetitive motions (e.g., in the elbow or shoulder).

- **Cartilage Damage**: May occur in the knee or shoulder due to improper movements or falls.

3. Recovery Strategies

A. Immediate First Aid (RICE):

- **Rest**: Stop any activity and rest the injured area.

- **Ice**: Apply ice packs for 15-20 minutes every hour to reduce swelling and pain.

- **Compression**: Use elastic bandages to compress the injured area, providing support and reducing swelling.

- **Elevation**: Elevate the injured area above heart level to reduce swelling.

B. Physical Therapy:

- **Rehabilitation Exercises**: Work with a physical therapist to develop a rehabilitation program that focuses on restoring strength, flexibility, and function.

- **Manual Therapy**: Consider techniques like massage or joint mobilization to promote healing and reduce pain.

C. Nutrition for Recovery:

- **Protein Intake**: Ensure adequate protein consumption to support muscle repair and recovery.

• **Anti-Inflammatory Foods**: Include foods rich in omega-3 fatty acids (salmon, walnuts), antioxidants (berries, leafy greens), and turmeric to help reduce inflammation.

D. Gradual Return to Training:

• **Consult a Professional**: Before returning to training, consult a healthcare provider or physical therapist to assess readiness.

• **Modify Intensity**: Begin with low-impact activities and gradually increase intensity based on comfort and recovery progress.

• **Focus on Technique**: During the return, prioritize proper technique to avoid re-injury.

4. Mental Recovery:

• **Mental Health**: Acknowledge the emotional impact of injuries. Engage in activities that promote mental well-being, such as mindfulness or relaxation techniques.

• **Goal Setting**: Set realistic rehabilitation goals to maintain motivation and a positive mindset during recovery.

Injury prevention and recovery are integral to a martial artist's training regimen. By implementing effective prevention strategies, understanding common injuries, and following a structured recovery plan, practitioners of Haidong Gumdo can reduce the risk of injuries and enhance their overall performance.

Continuous education about safe practices and regular consultation with instructors and healthcare professionals will further support a healthy and sustainable martial arts journey.

Conclusion

Practicing Haidong Gumdo is not only about mastering techniques and sparring but also about fostering a holistic approach to training that encompasses physical conditioning, nutrition, injury prevention, and mental resilience.

Key Takeaways:

- **Holistic Approach**: Integrating various aspects of training—strength, flexibility, cardiovascular conditioning, and mental focus—ensures a well-rounded martial artist who can perform effectively and safely.

- **Nutrition**: Proper nutrition fuels performance, aids recovery, and supports overall health. A balanced diet rich in macronutrients and micronutrients, along with adequate hydration, is essential for martial artists.

- **Injury Prevention**: Understanding common injuries and implementing strategies like proper warm-ups, technique mastery, and gradual progression can significantly reduce the risk of injuries.

- **Recovery**: Effective recovery strategies, including the RICE method, physical therapy, and nutrition for healing, are crucial for returning to training safely and quickly. Mental recovery is equally important, as it helps maintain motivation and mental well-being.

- **Continuous Learning**: Engaging with instructors, seeking feedback, and being open to learning will enhance not only technical skills but also overall understanding of martial arts principles.

By prioritizing these elements, practitioners of Haidong Gumdo can enjoy a rewarding martial arts journey, achieve their personal goals, and maintain longevity in their practice. Ultimately, the combination of physical skills, mental fortitude, and a commitment to health will lead to success both in the dojo and in everyday life.

Glossary Of Terms

Here's a glossary of key terms commonly used in Haidong Gumdo, along with their definitions:

- **Bong**: A traditional sword used in Haidong Gumdo, typically characterized by its curved blade.

- **Chigi**: A term referring to a strike or cut, usually executed with the sword.

- **Do**: Translates to "way" or "path," indicating the philosophical journey of a martial artist.

- **Gumdo**: Literally means "sword way," referring to the practice of swordsmanship as a martial art.

- **Hyung**: Forms or patterns that practitioners learn and practice to develop technique, timing, and movement.

- **Kihap**: A spirited shout or yell performed during techniques to focus energy and increase power.

- **Kwan**: A school or style within martial arts; can refer to the specific school of Haidong Gumdo.

- **Mugunghwa**: The national flower of Korea, often symbolizing resilience and determination in martial arts.

- **Paldan**: A stance or position that serves as a foundation for various techniques and movements.

- **Seon**: A state of mindfulness and mental clarity that practitioners strive to achieve during training.

- **Seon-ki**: The mental aspect of martial arts, emphasizing focus, discipline, and the cultivation of inner peace.

- **Sogi**: Refers to various stances used in Haidong Gumdo, each with specific applications for technique execution.

- **Sool**: Refers to techniques or skills, often focusing on specific movements or strikes.

- **Taeguk**: A symbol representing the balance of opposing forces, commonly used in Korean martial arts to convey philosophical principles.

- **Yeo**: The concept of fluidity or flexibility in movement, allowing practitioners to adapt and respond effectively.

- **Yeon**: Refers to the spirit or essence of martial arts training, emphasizing harmony between mind and body.

Haidong Gumdo practitioners can use this dictionary as a starting point for learning the language and principles of the art. Gaining familiarity with these terminology improves one's ability to communicate and understand the art's concepts and procedures, which in turn helps one feel more connected to the practice and its philosophical foundations.

ABOUT THE AUTHOR:

Kameron Jalen, an author, frequently employs his profound comprehension of human nature and personal experiences to investigate a diverse array of themes in his writing. His compositions may encompass instructional materials, non-fiction, or fiction, which demonstrate his capacity to articulate intricate concepts in a manner that is both engaging and comprehensible. Jalen's objective in his writing is to motivate and inspire readers by imparting knowledge on the significance of personal development, self-discipline, and resilience.

Kameron Jalen is also a dedicated martial arts practitioner, having trained in a variety of disciplines. His proficiency in martial arts is not only indicative of his physical abilities, but also underscores the philosophical and cerebral components of the discipline. He is likely to promote the advantages of martial arts in the development of focus, discipline, and confidence, and he may conduct seminars or teach classes to disseminate his expertise. He integrates the principles of hard work and perseverance into both his writing and teaching, as evidenced by his martial arts journey.

Kameron Jalen has a Ph.D. in a pertinent discipline from a prestigious university in the United States, in addition to his creative and physical activities. His academic education equips him with a robust foundation for his writing and teaching, enabling him to approach subjects with a critical and analytical perspective. His scholarly work and research may concentrate on the social implications of martial arts, human behavior, or psychology, thereby contributing to both academic discourse and practical applications.

Kameron Jalen possesses an uncommon combination of academic rigor, physical prowess, and creativity. He remains a source of inspiration and influence for those in his vicinity, motivating them to pursue their interests and aspire for excellence in all aspects of life because of his diverse talents. Jalen is dedicated to the promotion of personal and professional development, whether through his academic lectures, martial arts classes, or publications.

THE END